Feel good aging through

Make your 60s appear younger with these 22 proven tips

By

Dr mandy frankford

Feel good aging through

TABLE OF CONTENT

INTRODUCTION

How do you feel about becoming older?

Some people find it to be a frightening period of change and isolation.

Nevertheless, things don't have to be that way. That shouldn't, in actuality. We are social beings, and getting older is not something you do alone. That is the essence of positive aging.

The key to "aging gracefully" is how we define, perceive, and accept the changes.

expected adjustments that were unanticipated

You understand the ones I mean. "Oof," you say as you get out of a chair. "Oof," you say as you reach into a low cupboard for something. "Oof" as you stoop to put on your shoes.

Honestly, just getting out of bed in the morning requires a lot."Euuurgh-oooofff-ughhh-aargh... ohhh gawwwd," all while stretching your achy muscles, hurting back, stiff neck, and blinking your eyes because WHERE ARE MY GLASSES I CAN'T SEE, all at the same time.

That's it; stop letting me continue doing that old lady "oof" grunting, I yelled. Without all those geriatric noises coming from my cake-hole, I can stand up on my own just fine. (Keith is now strictly instructed to give me the

Pensioner Puffing look whenever I do it.)

To put it another way, becoming older can be a nuisance.

And I do mean it figuratively. I'm not quite 50 and

already I feel THIS sore! There are aches and pains you

never realized could possibly exist in one body.

That is to say, WHEN DID I GROW OLD? Why, then, was I

never informed of any of these things that would occur

as the years passed?

Naturally, I'm not implying that I don't enjoy getting

older. I do. I'm more self-assured, I love life, and I truly

love that I'm getting close to being 50 instead of 20. I

enjoy being the age I am in the modern world—young

enough to use and appreciate technology but old

enough to remember a period before it. Isn't that what

people who belong to Generation X say about us?

Anyway, that's me. I fall squarely in the middle of that appreciating spectrum.

But, I believe we should have some fun with it,No matter how hard we try to turn back the clock, that will happen to even the greatest among us. I'm not fighting against these flaws brought on by aging and the sagging of our bodies, but occasionally I do wish they would give us a little relief. I mean, is it Christmas again? ALREADY? Where did autumn go? I definitely closed my eyes too quickly and missed it AGAIN.

Just a little bit slower, Time. Ageing IS a privilege, but for goodness' sake, give me a minute so I can get my glasses and take it all in.

CHAPTER 1

The 18 worst things about aging that I just wasn't ready for are listed here for your pleasure.

1. Jowls

They advised against wrinkling! They advised using this

lotion to prevent deep wrinkles. I can put up with crow's

feet all day, but in my opinion, jowls are the most

detestable aspect of physical aging. I do not mind having

wrinkles; in fact, I rather enjoy them. The fine creases

around my eyes that Botox claims to eliminate are not

something I want (disclosure: I do have it on my

forehead, but only subtly). So would you kindly, kindly, kindly, stop sagging skin around my jawline? I'm tired of having a glum expression when I already know how to put on a resting bitch face thanks to years of practice. More motivation is not necessary.

2. Fuzzy facial hair

No one has ever said that as you age, your face will get increasingly puffy.When you're younger, you may believe that having all that fluffy down on your chin and cheeks is a characteristic of old ladies, but in actuality, you are at least 30–40 years younger than those ladies when the fluff is out in full force. I've managed to dodge the long, stray hairs on my chin thus far, but I predict they'll start to grow soon.

3. Retracting gums

I don't just happen to have excellent teeth at 49 years

old: I genuinely take care of them. Frequent flossing,

brushing, and dental exams; abstaining from smoking;

and consuming just a moderate amount of sugar,

alcohol, or coffee.

And I am aware that having children frequently damages

your teeth, therefore the fact that I have never had

children has contributed to my teeth continuing to be

strong and healthy But, OH MY GOD -My gums are

receding and I can't stop it. My teeth get even more

sensitive as a result. I just don't know how much further

they're going to withdraw before I develop the longest

gnashers in the entire world since I currently have all

teeth and almost no gum.

4. Aching knees

My knees constantly serve as a reminder that they are

no longer 20 years old.

You're rising from a squat, are you? Here's a quick sting.

Taking a run? Given that the right one was hurting

yesterday, we reasoned that the left one should be

hurting today. More than 30 seconds were spent lying

on the ground? While you get up from THAT posture,

LOL, let me stifle my laughter. Also, keep in mind that

your words, not ours, should always come first.

5. A dislike of current music

You WILL ask, "What IS this racket?" in regards to modern music, no matter HOW many times you tell yourself that you won't 'when you get old'. It is unavoidable. Only 5% of the performers nominated for The Brit Awards are known to me, and even that number is inflated by Annie Lennox odd nomination for Best Female Artist AGAIN AGAIN, which makes up 4% of the nominees. I always end myself asking, "Who? WHO?" after each name that is read. I can't help but claim it's simply "noise" if I happen to see the performers in action or hear a little piece of Radio 1 playing at some time during the day, And when you begin claiming that it wasn't like that "in my day" and that "music was proper music back then," you KNOW you have inexorably entered The Land of Decrepitness.

6. Unabated weight increase

At 45, your body experiences something... It attracts fat deposits, calories, and cellulite like a magnet. It seems that your body prefers to either 1. Put the question to you: Are you resistant to gaining weight? Shall we play a game to see how much weight you can hold off as I keep presenting you with new challenges to make staying in shape more difficult? or 2. Not seek your advice?at all and simply dump your metabolism in 2017 instead. Even though I made a vow to myself at the age of 30 that I wouldn't get bingo wings, I haven't yet figured out which one it is, but in the meantime I know that it's very hard to lose belly/thigh fat or avoid getting bingo wings.

Hahaha...

7. Diminished vision

I asked my mother, who was stretching out the soup

packet so far from her face to read it, when I was ten

years old, as we were shopping. Why is she making such

a strained, wide-eyed expression?

It's frustrating to lose your 20-20 vision. Fortunately, I

have amazing long vision, which makes everything,

except for the fact that I never notice where the year

has gone while driving, watching TV, and gazing out the

window, crystal clear for me [I'll tell you right now that

the only thing I never seem to notice is where the year

goes]. Yet, I'll be darned if I can read or concentrate on

anything within arm's reach without making my eyes

squint so much that you'd think I'd somehow figured out

where the last year had actually gone.

8. Elderly puffing

Introduction paragraph. Making the bed from scratch

and new? Oof. As you finish your downward-facing dog

yoga pose, do you stand up? Oof. picking up the bulky

laundry basket containing the damp clothes? Oof.

Pulling the large Instant Pot out of the cupboard's back?

Oh, oh, oh.

9. Skin coloration

If I could change the past and offer myself some advise

(for years, I had no idea what I'd say when I read such "If

you could"

Avoid sunbathing, FFS, if you could provide advice to

your younger self (ask yourself this question). The

regrettable after-effects are splashed all over my cheeks,

jawline, and down my neck even though I haven't

exposed my face to the sun in the manner of George

Hamilton in many years (if you just said "who?" then I'm

not sure why you're reading this, aside from future

research purposes). In my 20s, nobody ever advised me

to quit sunbathing or, worse, to stop using sunbeds. (I

am a nasty person, I realize that. I was, at least.) Perhaps

if I had told my mother I was using them, she might have

advised me to quit, but I believe I was aware of what I was doing. Hence, pigmentation of the skin is Totally preventable and caused by one's own actions.

10. Repeatedly thinking, "I'm old enough to be their mother,"

Although I'm easily old enough to be a grandmother and I AM actually old enough to have children, I still get utterly shocked when any youngish adult with a stable job and a mortgage could, quite easily - and without any sort of 80s or 90s era teenage shenanigans on my part - be my son or daughter. Have you ever heard a more acute case of age denial than that. When it comes to the whole "could I be their mother?" thing, I'm constantly wondering how I got to be this old.

11. Nighttime sweating

Oh, well, we can probably credit the Big M (or the Big Pre-M) for that. Either that, or my ability to estimate the quantity of bedding and linen my bed will require at any given time of year is seriously hampered. Perhaps, what's really occurred is that I've transformed into a human radiator with the dream talents of a really energetic party animal (with issues), a feat that would defy even big man Freud. Easily distracted? Let's take that and let it all out through your sweat glands during the night, shall we?

12. Pains, aches, and more pains

In my lifetime, I'm not sure if I'll ever have another

experience. Here is an example of a typical Day of Aches:

Who said anything hurtful? Well, my left knee hurts like

crazy, and then there's the pain running up and down

the back of my right leg because I believe I sat too long

in one position, and my neck hurts because I slept funny

last night, and oh, I forgot the sore joints in my two little

fingers that I can attribute to onset arthritis (because my

mum has bad arthritis), and I shouldn't pick up my tea

with my left hand because there's still some residual

tennis elbow pain there, and hey boy that plantar

fasciitis in my foot is acting up again, and I can't pick up

my tea with my left hand because of the lingering

discomfort in my left tennis elbow. Did I also mention

that my lower back pain started after I went to get my

wellies and hasn't subsided for many days?

13. The cliche that "policemen seem young" actually exists.

A few weeks ago, we got a brand-new vehicle. The

sweet young man who sold us the automobile told me

while I was completing the papers that he would be

celebrating his 21st birthday this coming weekend. What

Was I Doing When They Were Born? is a game that I

constantly play in my head, and I don't know about you..

And when you realize the salesman who sold you your

car was born in THIS century—that is, that his date of

birth begins with a 2 instead of a 1—you freak out. WHY

is he not attending class? WHY isn't his mother running

around seeking for him? WHY does he have a deep voice and the appearance of an adult man? WHY is he dressed professionally with a suit and tie? HOW did I figure out I passed my driving test 10 years before he was even born? WHY?

14. Calluses

This, however, is not at all what I anticipated. My bunions aren't that bad, but for some reason,

my TINY toes have developed strange little bunions that have expanded throughout the years to the point that they resemble horns on my baby toes. Even their name is endearing: bunionettes. Awwww.

You weird little devil toe horns, leave now.

15. Finding your birth year is a never-ending task

If you're filling out an online form, you'll need to scroll endlessly to find your birth year.

16. Aging hands and feet

Nearly as unpleasant as the jowl issue is the day you realize your hands have aged. Once more, I'm in my 40s, not old ladies, and I don't belong in that. And before I even begin, what's up with those venous feet? why are there so many veins? Who said they'd look odd and old? Nobody, to be precise.

17. Wanting to remain at home

I'm really horrified at the prospect of staying out past 11 o'clock. I used to go partying every week, leaving the house at 10 p.m. to take the train from Clapham Junction into central London and arrive at the club at around 11 p.m. (and be one of the early ones). Moreover, on a Friday night, after a long day of standing up all day at work in retail? I don't understand how I could EVER THINK about doing that right now, let alone POSSIBLY consider it. At 10 p.m., I want to be reading my email instead of going outside At 10 o'clock at night, I want to make sure the front door is closed, make "one final cup of tea," and, perhaps, remember to turn on the electric blanket at least an hour earlier.

18. The speed at which time flies

Just ten years have passed since the century, not twenty.

TWENTY YEARS*, let it sink in. Just how is that possible?

I just don't get it. Marty went back in time only 30 years

in Back to the Future, which was released 36 years ago.

Goddammit, the age of Macaulay Culkin is 41.As with

the time interval between 1939 and 1980, the time

interval between 1980 and now is also equal. Why,

exactly? Who was responsible for this? How on earth is

it already 2023?How long ago was 2020? 2015 wasn't

that long ago, was it? WHO is tampering with the idea of

time and space? I've been considering this... I'm

mistaken; the millennium will have passed twenty-three

years ago in less than six weeks.

CHAPTER 2

. *How will you make plans and get ready for the coming years of your life?*

The key is attitude. No matter how old you are, having a bad attitude can only make your experience worse. There is more to healthy aging than "roses and daffodils." Ageing can be challenging and unpleasant at times. Yet, research demonstrates that how we choose to respond to the terrible events in our life has a

significant impact.

Note that at the beginning of this chapter I asked?How

will you organize and get ready for the coming years of

your life? Some people prefer not to plan so far ahead.

Others are moving in that direction already.We will

certainly get at our destination eventually. We may

either force ourselves to do it or do it in total denial.

Instead, we might embrace the third act, enjoy ourselves

a little, and end up in the grave exhausted.Life is a

banquet, and most of the poor suckers are starving to

death, to quote Auntie Mamie in her classic words.It can

be challenging to accept aging. It's possible that our

body can no longer perform the functions it did when

we were kids or younger. Bones are more brittle. Aches

and pains can occur frequently.We experience eyesight loss. Our hair turns white or gray. It can come out at times. Our ears and noses enlarge. We become smaller. We are psychologically affected by these events. This is especially true in societies where elders are not revered.We struggle to find our position as we become older and lose value in our society. We must redefine who we are and decide on our mission. Poor mental health is also a result of loneliness and loss of independence.The daily tasks that older persons used to complete on their own may now require assistance. Family tensions and frustration may result from this. Another fact of aging is losing a life partner. A person may experience any of these things, along with others.

The basic conclusion is that as we get older, we can still learn complex jobs and retain that knowledge just as well as a younger individual. Crystallized intelligence is advantageous to older people as well. This is the capacity to apply knowledge that has been acquired and experience to solve new issues. Age increases this type of intelligence.

Growing older brings about changes in a variety of areas, including the physical, mental, social, emotional, and sexual. You might view some of these changes as favorable and others as negative. The tip is to take proactive measures to maintain your health and reduce the negative effects of aging while maximizing the positive aspects.

Feel good aging through

CHAPTER 3

This is what comes to your mind when aging. As follows:

1. Everyone anticipates dying.

Older folks start to withdraw from their networks as a result of their acceptance that they are aging and losing abilities.

2. Fewer interactions allow for more behavioral freedom.

As a result, their behavior takes on a "I can do whatever I want" attitude.

3. Men and women experience things differently.

Males play crucial roles. Ladies don't.

4. The ego changes with age.

The older adult makes way so the younger one can fill

the role they are leaving.

The senior looks for personal enjoyment.

5. Total disengagement happens whenever society is ready for it.

Only when society is ready for it can older persons

transition.

6. If employees lose their roles, disengagement may result.

Gender has an impact on roles. Labor is performed by men. Women are in charge of household duties. Disengagement occurs if they are unable to carry out their responsibilities.

7. Societal acceptance is a function of readiness.

When an older adult begins thinking their mortality, experience a loss of prestige, and lose "ego energy," then society enables disengagement.

8. Relational incentives grow more varied.

Upward mobility is frequently included in societal rewards. Horizontal rewards result from disengagement.

To fill the vertical reward hole, people turn to their remaining interpersonal connections.

9. Its theory transcends cultural boundaries..

It adopts the social customs of the individual. The entire procedure is agreeable to both the individual and society. When someone disengages depends on how useful they are. If society still finds the person to be helpful, disengagement is delayed.

Those with a different viewpoint emphasize youth and physical attractiveness over the wisdom that might come with experience. This group frequently makes the decision to combat aging.

Aging is a given. Although we all know this to be true, as you read more, you'll discover that some individuals think aging is an illness. They think it is treatable.

The capacity of an individual to preserve continuity between who they were and who they are becoming as they age, including their habits, interests, lifestyle, and connections. Similar to the idea of intelligence that has solidified.A person applies what they have learned from the past to changes that will occur in the future.

Living your best life and being in good bodily and mental health are the keys to aging gracefully. It's not about trying to appear like you're in your 20s. If you take good care of yourself, you can age like a fine wine.

CHAPTER 4

Make your 60s appear younger with these 22 proven tips

Aging is a mental battle over physical challenges, just like everything else.

While it's true that we can't stop some chronic illnesses by keeping a positive mindset, it's also true that by doing so, we can make the aging process much more pleasant and civil. If you want to improve your quality of life as a senior,

Here are twenty two clever ideas to help a senior, or a senior's loved one, improve outlook and lead a happier, healthier lifetime.

1. Elderly experience a sense of life "passing them by."

Seniors frequently believe they are no longer relevant. In many circumstances, a senior's spouse has passed away, and the person's social connections may not be as strong as they once were.

Elderly persons can easily experience depression in these situations or feel abandoned and forgotten.

Fortunately, not every senior has to assume this.

Instead, it is simple to overcome this "disadvantage" by making sure that senior citizens are included in family get-together, social events, and neighborhood activities. This helps to promote the growth of new relationships and experiences while also assisting in the fight against emotions of loneliness.

2. It can be challenging to date

Encourage senior citizens to join clubs, groups, and organizations that share their interests. Dating at 70 may be different than it was at 17, but it's still very possible, and many seniors discover that they genuinely love dating later in life.

3. Seniors frequently feel exhausted and worn out

 While it's typical for older folks to feel less active and outgoing than they once did, it's not reasonable to expect to spend every waking hour in seclusion as a result. Seniors can increase their energy by exercising, eating a good diet, lots of sound sleep, and socializing with family and friends. A visit to the doctor may be necessary if you experience persistent fatigue because some supplements may help you feel more energized.

4. Physical activity and exercise may be challenging or painful.

Seniors need to continue being active to maintain their health. Sadly, as we get older, things get harder and harder. Seniors just need to modify their level and type of activity to maintain the cardiovascular system, joints, and bones in good health and function without being overexercised.

According to scientific research, those who regularly engage in physical activity not only live longer but also may do so in a better way, with more years spent free from illness or injury.

In a study of persons aged 40 and older, walking 8,000 steps or more per day was linked to a 51% lower risk of death from all causes than walking only 4,000 steps. By engaging in physical activity throughout the day, such as gardening, walking the dog, and choosing the stairs over the elevator, you can boost the amount of steps you take each day.

Feel good aging through

For instance, water aerobics, yoga, or swimming may be the best options for a senior who once enjoyed long distance running but now finds it challenging. While many seniors believe that being older means they can no longer lead active lifestyles, it's more common that a simple change is all that's required.

5. It's common for seniors to struggle with their sense of attractiveness.

Age-related changes to the body and appearance are inevitable, but seniors don't have to experience self-consciousness as a result. Many seniors discover that going to the salon or indulging in self-care or beauty rituals (such as facials, massages, or pedicures) that they couldn't justify when they were younger are all fantastic ways to feel more appealing.

6. The elder can feel "out of touch" with the times.

Solution: Seniors frequently misunderstand Justin Bieber and The Kardashians. Fortunately, seniors can easily feel more active and engaged by either learning more about contemporary pop culture or hanging out with people who value the same historical periods and recollections as they do.

senior citizens who don't like reading pop culture publications periodicals would appreciate participating in themed events or getting together with pals to reminisce about the good old days.

Feel good aging through

7. Driving may become challenging or forbidden

The loss of some privileges, like driving, is among the things seniors fear aging most. Some seniors may inevitably lose their driving rights, but this doesn't necessarily mean that they will lose the ability to take care of themselves.

In reality, seniors who are unable to drive have a variety of transportation options. Public transportation may be a wise choice in many situations. In other circumstances, a senior may appreciate taking a shuttle that is designated for elders and that helps them do tasks like shopping.

Seniors may even decide to take a pleasant, unhurried stroll to their destination. While the correct response will vary based on a senior's health and energy levels, turning older should not entail a complete loss of freedom.

8. Missing family members might make you lonely

Being separated from family and friends is a problem that many seniors face. However, regular phone calls, Skype sessions, and handwritten letters may help bridge even the biggest physical distances and guarantee joyful, intimate connections between seniors and their families.

9. Elderly are frequently bored with their daily activities.

Truth be told, growing older can be dull. Fortunately, elders can avoid ennui by enrolling in an art class, attending a local university program on an audit basis, volunteering or acquiring new knowledge. Even if old age comes with many difficulties, it also provides a certain amount of free time that enables seniors to fully benefit from chances and improve themselves in a variety of ways.

10. It can be challenging to locate clothes that an elderly person enjoys.

Many senior citizens discover that their past fashion preferences don't fit well with their current lifestyles as they get older. Fortunately, this only requires some adaptation. It may not be possible for seniors to wear the flaring dresses or handsome suits they once loved, but it is simple to discover clothing that a senior enjoys and feels comfortable in. Maybe just a quick trip to the store is needed!

11. Elderly are not accustomed to the quick-paced nature of the modern world Solution:

Slow down. Seniors have a reason to be a little worried by how rapidly time has passed, and it may be in both of our best interests to slow down and be more deliberate while spending time with them. We have the time and flexibility when we're not in a hurry or hustling to appreciate our encounters with the elder instead of

rushing through them.

12. Elderly frequently feel unwell.

Solution: Seniors with ailments that may be managed

with diet, exercise, or medication frequently feel better

after receiving the right care. While it's unreasonable for

many seniors to think they'll be as active at 80 as they

were at 20, there's also no reason to assume that

becoming older has to entail constantly feeling unwell.

13. Elderly find it challenging to adapt to advancing years.

Assist the elderly person in realizing that aging has

many positive aspects and that every stage of life is

lovely. While many seniors find it difficult to accept their aging, recognizing the truths of it and embracing the next stage gracefully makes the entire process simpler to endure for seniors.

14. sleeping well at night

You can stay healthy and alert by getting adequate sleep. Even though they require the same seven to nine hours of sleep as other adults, older folks frequently fall short of this requirement. Sleeping may be made more difficult by illness or pain, and some medications may keep you awake. Without enough sleep, a person may become agitated, unhappy, forgetful, and more susceptible to accidents such as falls.

In a study of persons over 65, it was discovered that those who slept poorly had a harder time concentrating and solving problems than those who slept well.

Another study, which examined data from about 8,000 individuals, revealed that those in their 50s and 60s who slept six hours or less every night had a higher chance of acquiring dementia in later life.

15. Stop smoking.

Research shows that stopping smoking will improve your health regardless of your age or length of smoking, even if you're 60 years old or older and have been a smoker for many years.

 If you stop smoking at any age, you'll reduce your risk of developing cancer, heart disease, stroke, and lung disease, improve your blood circulation, boost your senses of taste and smell, and be a healthy role model for others.

One study indicated that smokers were three times more likely to pass away within a six-year follow-up period than non-smokers among men and women aged 55 to 74 and 60 to 74, respectively.

16. substances like alcohol

Elderly people should abstain from or consume alcohol in moderation, just like all adults. Age-related social and physical changes can, in fact, increase an older person's susceptibility to alcohol misuse and abuse as well as their vulnerability to its negative effects. dependency on alcohol or heavy intake affects Every organ in the body, including the brain, is impacted by alcoholism or severe drinking. According to a thorough study by the National Institute on Alcohol Abuse and Alcoholism, alcohol consumption is rising among older persons, particularly women. Also, the researchers discovered proof that both alcohol-dependent men and women exhibit indicators of early aging in specific brain regions. Also, older persons who drink heavily and for an extended period of time may have poorer heart health. These studies indicate that reducing or quitting alcohol use may benefit heart health and delay the accelerated aging associated with heavy alcohol use.

17. keeping your mental health in check

To maintain total wellness and a high standard of living, you must maintain good mental health. As a result, It has an impact on our decisions, actions, and interactions with others. Healthy aging depends on controlling social isolation, loneliness, stress, sadness, and mood through medical treatment and self-care.

18. Isolation from others and loneliness

Maintaining social relationships can be challenging as people age due to factors including hearing and vision loss, memory loss, disability, trouble getting about, and the loss of relatives and friends. Because of this, older persons are more likely to experience social isolation or loneliness. Despite their similar sounds, loneliness and social isolation are not the same. Social isolation, on the other hand, refers to a lack of social contacts and having few individuals to frequently communicate with. Loneliness is the uncomfortable sense of being alone or isolated.

19. Hobbies and recreational pursuits

Your favorite activities may benefit your health in addition to being enjoyable. According to research, those who engage in hobbies, social activities, and other leisure-time pursuits may have a lower risk of developing certain health issues. A community choir program for older individuals, for instance, was proven to minimize loneliness and boost interest in life, according to one study. Another study found that older persons who read for at least one hour each day or participate in other hobbies had a lower risk of dementia

than those who read for less than 30 minutes each day.

20. Stay in Your Day Job

Early retirement may not be the greatest option for your

health, unless you have a fulfilling second career.

According to the Longevity Project study, those who put

in a lot of effort at a profession they like live the longest.

That could be the secret to staying around for a while,

combined with having nice friends and a happy marriage.

21. Self-Assurance

According to studies, self-esteem rises as you get older

and rises with wealth, education, good health, and work.

But after 60 it starts to decline. That might be the case

as people start to experience health problems and look for new callings after retiring. We might observe that change as a result of longer life expectancy, healthier lifestyles, and later retirement.

22. The Skin

Everyone has witnessed the "age spots" or "liver spots" that can appear after years in the sun.

It becomes more difficult for your skin to retain moisture as you age and wrinkle, which can result in dry, itchy skin. As you age, you lose soft tissue, which makes veins more noticeable. In your hands, this is especially true. Use broad-spectrum sunscreen with a minimum SPF of 30 to shield your hands from the sun's rays.

For gardening or cleaning, put on cotton-lined gloves

and use a light soap or cleanser that won't remove your

hands' natural oils. Moisturizers and a nutritious diet

with lots of vitamins, antioxidants, and omega-3 fatty

acids also can help keep your skin and nails healthy.

CHAPTER 5

The benefits of aging

This is a list of 10 positive elements of becoming older, including both financial and personal benefits.

1. A More Positive Perspective

It may come as a surprise to some, but studies have

shown that seniors are among the happiest age groups,

and that they are substantially happier than their middle-aged peers. Dr. Saverio Strange, the study's author, speculates that this may be related to improved coping skills. Elderly adults typically possess internal defenses that enable them to handle hardship or adverse conditions better than younger people." The fact that older people are "more comfortable being themselves" is another factor that may contribute to their happiness.

2. Grandkids

Gore Vidal, a writer from the United States, once joked, Have only grandchildren; never have children.

Grandparents frequently get to share in the delights of

young children without having to deal with diaper

changes and restless nights.

When grandparents show their love to their grandkids, it

warms their hearts and has a positive impact on the

recipients of that love. According to research, children

require four to six involved, nurturing adults in their lives

in order to completely develop emotionally and socially,

and the parent-child relationship and the grandparent-

grandchild relationship are the two relationships that

have the most emotional impact on children.

3. More Time with Family and Friends

Retirement is not inherently enjoyable or restful; rather,

what is done with that time to make it special. Spending

time with family, friends, and other loved ones is one of the finest aspects of retirement.

4. Possibility of Pursuing Your Goals

George Elliot, a writer of Victorian novels "It's never too late to be what you may have become," the Victorian author George Elliot once penned. Retirement is a great opportunity to pursue passions and aspirations that you may have put on hold. You may, for instance, pick up a new language, go on the vacation of a lifetime, or pen the book that has been waiting to be written in your thoughts.

5. Civic involvement and volunteer work

Getting older gives one a sense of a larger perspective, and it frequently leads people to be more motivated to devote a large portion of their time and energy to improving and fostering a better environment for future generations. Seniors who have retired have greater time for civic engagement in addition to time with loved ones, pursuing passions, and personal goals. Seniors who have retired have more time to participate in politics and civic affairs, and they do so. For instance, figures from the U.S. Census Bureau show that voters over 65 vote at a higher rate than voters of any other age group. They also contribute to volunteering a lot. One-fourth of American seniors 65 and older engaged in volunteer work in 2015, according to the Bureau of Labor and Statistics.

6. Wisdom

A Smithsonian magazine article summarized a number of recent studies showing the advantages of aging on the mind and emotions. Seniors have better emotional regulation than those of different ages, according to a study mentioned in the article. A gambling game "intended to generate regret" was played by participants of all ages by researchers, and they discovered that "unlike 20-somethings,

People in their 60s didn't cry over losses and weren't as likely to try to make up for them by subsequently taking significant risks.

7. More Empathy and Improved Social Skills

Participants in a another study, also cited in the aforementioned article, were asked for suggestions for fictitious " Dear Abby " letter writers. The results showed that elders have stronger social and compassionate skills. According to the study, older subjects performed better than younger ones at imagining several points of view, formulating numerous alternatives, and suggesting compromises. Even though elders may have more developed social abilities than their younger counterparts, they are nonetheless prone to loneliness.

8. Social Security, Medicare, and Guaranteed Minimum Income

In a piece on the history of aging, we talked about how, prior to the 20th century, elderly people without the means to support themselves were compelled to live in institutions known as "workhouses" or "poorhouses." Seniors without family members who could take care of them or who are not independently rich have to deal with this. Even though senior poverty is still a significant issue, Medicaid and Social Security ensure that all American seniors have access to a minimum guaranteed income and health insurance, regardless of their wealth or the presence of dependent children. "We can never insure one-hundred percent of the population," said President Franklin D. Roosevelt in 1935, referring to the significance of Social Security and other safety-net programs that he helped put into place."We will never be able to completely protect the populace from all of

the risks and vicissitudes of life. Nonetheless, we have

made an effort to create a legislation that would provide

some level of protection to the typical citizen and his

family against the loss of a job and against a life of abject

poverty.

9. Senior Discount

Although while senior discounts may seem insignificant,

there was probably a moment when you envied them.

People can save money by taking advantage of the

discounts available to seniors during a time when

income is frequently fixed and constrained. These

reductions are a terrific incentive for seniors to take use of their retirement because they frequently apply to the services that keep them active and interested.

These reductions also give seniors a fantastic incentive to enjoy their retirement because they frequently apply to the things that keep seniors interested and active, like transportation, amusement, and entertainment.

10. Feeling of Achievement

Elderly folks frequently possess a positive sense of accomplishment-based pride. These successes don't have to be enormous feats. A working class hero is something to be, as John Lennon sang in the song. The basis of a happy fulfillment in old life can be laid by seemingly unremarkable accomplishments like raising a healthy and happy kid, being happily married, participating in the nation's defense, or retiring from a job in good standing after years of devoted service.